Baby Boomers
BE AWARE! ™

Vital Knowledge for
Boomers and their Parents
featuring
Essential, Informative, Cautionary,
Life-Saving and Spiritually-Uplifting
Messages, True Stories, Stats, Checklists,
and Insights to Help Save Time, Energy and
Money to Achieve and Maintain Everyone's
"Health and Safety"

by
Edward R. Williams

ISBN-13: 978-1456338329
SBN-10: 1456338323

All Design, Art and Branding by ERW
Copyright © 2011 by ERW

Dedicated to my
Mother-In-Law

Baby Boomers
BE AWARE! ™

CONTENTS

PREFACE

Initially this was to be a book of caution and information for Baby Boomers facing the many responsibilities of Parent healthcare issues, but as I began documenting my experiences I realized that the subject matter takes on an ironic cycle. Since we are in line for what our parents are, or will be, experiencing; this information actually portends our future, *and our childrens' future*.

Although painful to re-live and document I felt that my experiences needed to be told because for the first time I truly understood that seemingly trite statement; "If this information can prevent even one person from going through what I experienced then it will have been worth the effort".

INTRODUCTION

Are you one of the 78 million Baby-Boomers who will become eligible for Social Security in the near future?   This is a scary history-making statistic especially when you consider that as of mid-2009 Social Security has been evaluated to go insolvent - that is, run out of funds entirely - in 2037, that's 4 years earlier than previously predicted. Scarier is that Medicare goes insolvent as soon as 2017 that's 2 years earlier than previously predicted. These facts are according to the Treasury Department and the Health and Human Services Department.

The vast percentage of Baby-Boomers who have one or more Parent facing healthcare issues may someday need to consider alternative living conditions for them such as assisted living in their own home or living out their remaining years in any of the various convalescent, rehabilitation, nursing, or senior facilities.   While this can be a truly traumatic life change for them, it will also touch on and affect the lives of Boomers and their siblings as well as their families.

What you are about to read throughout is a true story.   Let my pain be your gain.

SAVE THE LIFE OF YOUR PARENT!
True Life Present Day Cautionary Story #1

My mother-in-law, a truly dear lady in all respects, broke her hip at age 83. She owned no property nor had any assets. Her three Baby Boomer children who loved her dearly were not in a financial position to afford 24 hour care for her in her rented home. Being a member of Christian Science she requested to go to one of their nursing homes in Southern California for rehabilitation and miraculously healed herself - *completely* - the bone fused correctly and fairly quickly; a true testament to her faith. But even though she physically healed, it was apparent that she was not up to the normal responsibilities of her former lifestyle.

Her children sought alternatives for her that would require fewer of those responsibilities and did the only thing they knew of at the time and turned to a 'Leisure World' styled community. Even though she already had friends there; the location was far away from family and the daily independent living that she so cherished was not working out as planned and was no longer an option for her.

It is at this point that Boomer decision-making for their parents' healthcare gets tough.

We were all novices from the beginning of this 'senior healthcare' journey. A decision had to be made to establish suitable living with less responsibility for her and under comfortable conditions which would also fit the budget. Thankfully a much closer geographical arrangement was reached in a senior facility complex in a city nearby us, where she could be visited and monitored frequently by all family members. This was our first regret though, that we didn't find her a place closer originally.

During this period I was very deep in my career as an artist working out of my home studio. I faced and met demanding daily, weekly and monthly deadlines while doing my best work late at night into early morning. This schedule allowed me the ability to visit my mother-in-law regularly during the day or early evening.

My income at that time was such that it also allowed me to complement her Social Security payment for her rent at the senior facility. I was happy to be in a position to financially help and did so with absolutely no thought of compensation. Money and the material world have never been what drive me; creativity, imagination and the quest for knowledge has. I have always seen money as a tool; a tool to accomplish things in life and to maintain basic survival needs.

So, this arrangement was successful until within the year she unfortunately fell once again and broke her other hip. While the Christian Science nursing home was again initially considered, the drive to visit and monitor her was deemed just too far away to repeat the whole process again. The trade-off of seeing her every day or every other day verses once a week at the most, helped in the decision. So in late 2000 the three siblings opted for what they could only believe in at the time to be a 'nice' nursing home for her to reside in while she 'rehabilitated' - I put quotes around these two words 'nice' and 'rehabilitated' as our experience would teach us, and as we would soon find out, both were nearly impossible to achieve in nursing/convalescent home environments.

The eldest male Boomer, a true brother, lived

back East and had a highly successful design business which unfortunately suffered from the fallout of Reaganomics. The other male Boomer, my wife's twin, another true brother, lived considerably far enough away that it was an effort to visit. He had a demanding job and family with children of his own to support, but he still made regular visits. Since my wife and I lived much closer we could visit a few times each week.

Admittedly we didn't do our homework and therefore we were unprepared and naïve about this next phase of the healthcare situation; so let our experience prevent you from having to endure the following trauma and heartbreak.

Through the Medicare system, convalescent facilities accommodate scheduled sessions by doctor-requested therapists to aid in 'rehabilitating' the injured with the objective that they will return to their previous lives. This is a blatant falsehood. The problem and reason is that therapy sessions consist of fifteen minutes to a half-hour *at most* about twice a week; so without a daily assist in this endeavor, it literally does no good. Instead, it actually perpetuates non-rehabilitation and here's why; unlike the peace of mind of being in their own homes with the ease of a low bed-to-floor ratio to assist and encourage them in their rehabilitation on a daily basis –they are instead in railed beds high off the floor with no opportunity to continue therapy on their own. Add to this the alien and ever increasing 'hospital' atmosphere and they can actually forget the reason they are there! This leads down a slippery slope whereby fragile minds begin to lose grasp of reality and therefore rehabilitation becomes next to impossible. This is a trap from which statistics show there is no escape.

Even though the location and environment of the facility was pleasant, with most hospital-like rooms surrounding a small park-like open air center with grassy lawns, flowers and trees as well as a friendly staff; we still dreaded seeing her in this thinly-disguised hospital. The heart-breaking fact that she was no longer in the familiar surroundings of her home but instead in an elevated bed in a room with several women she didn't know who were in various stages of mental-disorientation was just devastating. Yet we still believed at that point that she would rehabilitate as before and took the whole convalescent home rehabilitation environment for granted and assumed that all was well – it wasn't.

After daily visits turned into a month we began to notice that she was verbally communicating less and less. This was puzzling and only traumatized my wife even more than she already was. We were under the assumption that she was just tired or that we were catching her at a less than talkative time. Still it seemed strange; here she was in a nursing home for a broken hip – that's right a broken hip - and now she was hardly able to communicate! Soon this progressed to a state where she could hardly communicate at all. We demanded to see her doctor and upon arrival to confer with him we were notified that she had been rushed to the hospital with a severe case of dehydration and impaction, both so severe that the attending Hospital Doctor said it was the worst case he had ever seen!

This toxic combination of dehydration and impaction has an effect on muscles and especially on speech. Because of this neglect she lost the ability to swallow solid foods and required a stomach tube for food – for the rest of her life!

I still get painful shudders of anger and remorse from this insane outcome.

My wife loved her mother dearly and was shocked, horrified, devastated and in a severe nervous breakdown condition and I was blood-boiling furious, so at our wit's end we contacted lawyers to see what we could do about this criminal neglect issue. Astonishingly, we were informed by several lawyers that handled convalescent home neglect law suits that it was difficult to win cases against nursing homes because they are essentially "where people go to die".   This quote was their foregone matter- of-fact response.

We were outraged, mad, sad, traumatized, stressed and felt guilty as anyone could imagine because now along with the accompanying insanity she could only watch others' food delivered as she was fed by a tube, it was horrific and unbelievable. It literally became a form of madness for all concerned.

She could only communicate through nods and the joining of several words, but rarely sentences. From this point on her quality of life took on one long slow negative descent.

The only thing left was to see that she was as comfortable and comforted as much as possible under these surreal conditions.

Once a month she was treated to live music in the facility's community hall by a talented senior husband and wife musician team that played and sang 1930s and 1940s music. She really enjoyed those little concerts and would comment as best she could with, "Wonderful, just wonderful!" It was a source of joy she and I looked forward to in an otherwise daily state of hell on earth.

It was during one of those concerts that I noticed a woman in a wheelchair facing a side wall oblivious to the music. A nurse/caregiver came in and turned her wheelchair toward the stage, it was then that I saw who it was - it was a woman who was initially in the room with my mother-in-law at the very beginning of her admittance. She was much younger, probably in her 60s, who was bright, cheerful and talkative and who was there also to 'rehabilitate' from a broken hip. But how could this be? She was now a vegetable and it had only been a matter of a few months – how could she have declined to this state? I was shocked! I then had one of those epiphany moments; I realized what these homes really accomplished – *the exact opposite of what their names jointly stood for:* rehabilitation.

To prove my point further, a very close friend in his mid-to-late 60s, who lives on the east coast, woke up one morning paralyzed from the waist down. A totally bizarre situation to be sure, but to make a long story short, after several years he's able to walk with a cane and is nearly back to normal but initially he too was in a rehabilitation home. One day, fairly soon after he was admitted I spoke with him on the phone and he became distracted by the literal insanity around him to the point that I had to verbally snap him out of it, and this is a man who is incredibly bright and alert, but even he too began to succumb to the psychosis of that kind of environment. I immediately told him to get out of there, right then, at all costs; he understood, agreed and did.

These 'rehabilitation' centers are like any other business and while outwardly they are perceived as providing a service that projects rehabilitation as its goal, inwardly they know that standard operating procedures prevent that goal and that they are an 'industry of maintenance' at best. It is a fact that the high percentages of people who enter nursing homes do experience this as their final place of residence and thus are seen by the 'home' industry as a guaranteed source of income for the rest of their lives.

And such was the fate of my mother-in-law. After three years of the heart-rending horror of watching this dear lady slowly deteriorate the family reached a point of agreement that the only loving course to take was to let her go hospice-style. She died in the 'nice' nursing home.

So, if you have to put your parent in any of these homes; closely monitor their hydration levels and bowel movements. These are the two most important and proven susceptible issues for elderly victims of this system and are noted again in detail in the Checklist Section of this book. Obviously you cannot monitor them yourself on a daily basis which is why you need to check with the staff as they are *required* to keep a record of the amount of liquid your parent drinks and of the bowel movements they make daily. We were totally unaware of the potential severity and consequences of these issues. *Now you know.*

This knowledge extends to you Baby Boomers too. Someday, if you're not fortunate enough to be spared a life sentence in a 'nice' asylum, you now know what awaits you and the horror that you may face, as no one is exempt. Rich or poor, the money will be paid by you or by Social Security - or not, but the outcome will be the same.

How ironic for us Baby Boomers that Pete Townshend's iconic lyrics to the Who's rock classic "My Generation" would have such a deeper meaning.

HEALTHCARE STATISTICS

According to recent studies and statistics, the American Association of Homes and Services for the Aging (AAHSA) and MetLife estimate the US national average yearly cost for a patient in a healthcare/convalescent/nursing home facility in 2006 was $75,000.00. Patients who have assets, who own property or own their own home are subject for payment of these amounts.

For patients who have no assets, ultimately Medicare (Medicaid) will pay these costs, but still requires the signing-over of their monthly Social Security checks as co-pay for the total monthly/ yearly nursing home care payment.

The rate of patients discharged from hospitals but who still needed some sort of in-home health-care increased 53 percent (from 2 million to 4 million) between 1997 and 2006, according to the latest News and Numbers from the AHRQ (Agency for Healthcare Research and Quality).

There was a 30 percent increase (from 4 million to 5 million) in the rate of patients discharged to nursing homes or rehabilitation facilities during the same period.

In California in 2005, the average cost to maintain a patient per year in a nursing home/ rehabilitation facility was $77,000.00.

In 2006, the average daily nursing home costs for a semi-private room in Los Angeles, California was $180.00.

Nursing home and assisted living rates rose significantly from 2009 to 2010, according to the Market Survey of Long-Term Care Costs. Private room nursing home rates rose 4.6% to $229 per day or $83,585 per year, while assisted living rose 5.2% on average to $3,293 per month, or $39,516 per year. These increases come on top of increases from 2008 to 2009 when both nursing home and assisted living costs were up 3.3%.

In 2001, the number of deaths in nursing homes increased 66% over the past decade. People are going into nursing homes older, nursing home administrators say, *"Nursing homes get reimbursed at a higher rate for patients who require greater care, including those closer to death. [Nursing homes] are choosing the people who are more likely to die."*

HEALTHCARE CHECK LIST
The Essential Top Ten

1. COMPILE IMPORTANT PAPERS

Be prepared. Locate your parent's *original* birth certificates, photo I.D. (driver's license, passport), Social Security card, medical insurance policy, life insurance policy, and so on. Stored or filed in one safe place will insure peace of mind if and when any future medical or healthcare issues arise where they will be needed, and they will be needed.

2. RESEARCH ALL LOCAL SENIOR FACILITIES

If you have no choice other than this route to care for your parent; then take the time to research any of those facilities that are local to you. There are more being built everyday; there were two built within the last several years that are literally within a mile of my house and both are fully functional with no vacancies. There are probably several conveniently close to your location which will help to make the whole experience easier and at least less time-consuming as far as a commute is concerned.

For further in-depth local and regional senior healthcare information spend a leisurely afternoon searching the internet. You can access many helpful websites by entering these subjects in your browser's search field; senior healthcare, in-home caregivers, convalescent and/or nursing homes, senior services (day care, meals on wheels, city ride, etc.), aging in place, senior assisted living, Social Security, Medicare, and any other subject keywords pertinent to your situation.

3. BEWARE OF THE BROKEN HIP

This is the gateway to a potential downward spiral in which there is no turning back. As my experience clearly shows, and as difficult as it may seem to believe; a broken hip followed by the necessary rehabilitation process oftentimes can have a far worse effect than cancer recovery where the psyche of the patient is concerned. Nearly every tragic story I have heard during my education on this subject has started with a parent who broke their hip. It is a laborious and lengthy recovery process, in which true rehabilitation is rarely successful or even possible in a convalescent environment where the outcome instead becomes an almost unavoidable descent into psychosis, memory loss and alienation from even their family.

You or your parent's money used as a tool to insure home-environment stability for true rehabilitation is actually the supreme gift for health, safety and concern of a parent.

Any effort to allow rehabilitation in a parent's own home or familiar surroundings should be taken. It will greatly facilitate a quicker recovery and possibly add many more years to their life.

4. MONITOR FLUID INTAKE

Elderly people are especially prone to dehydration due to physiologic changes in the body related to the aging process. The aging brain isn't able to effectively determine how much water the body needs.

Seniors who live alone, are in the hospital, are recovering from major surgery, are disabled, have arthritis, suffer from Alzheimer's *and patients who live in nursing homes* are at the highest risk for dehydration.

Signs and symptoms of dehydration include irritability, confusion, rapid heart rate, decreased urine output, dry skin, constipation, fecal impaction, decreased blood pressure, and dizziness. In fact, dizziness caused by dehydration is often a contributing factor to falls by the elderly, which then commonly results in a broken hip.

So as you now can see it is a vicious cycle of; dehydration which could lead to dizziness, a fall and a broken hip OR a broken hip which could lead to dehydration which can then lead to a multitude of serious medical problems, which include coma, *organ failure* and eventual death.

Prevention is the first step in treating this condition. Make sure that fluids are readily available and monitor your parent to make sure they are drinking the liquids they are given. Adequate fluid intake is essential as part of preventative health care.

5. MEDICINE PRESCRIPTIONS AND DOSAGES

Both of these topics can create stressful issues on many fronts for both Boomer and Parent; hopefully the following tips will help alleviate some of them.

First, I would suggest that you purchase the organizational flip-top pill box 'medicine trays' that have the day of the week embossed and/or labeled on the top of each lid. These are available at most pharmacies and drug stores and you may need more than one to accommodate each different medicine's dosages.

   This will be a team effort if you employ a caregiver and even if not it is imperative to start out involving your parent to know which pills, how much and how many of each, and at what times they are required to take them. Writing this all down on a large calendar in clear view certainly helps as well. In most cases if you are lucky the doses will be whole pills, if not, you may have to halve or even quarter them. Be prepared to use a single edge razor with a sheet of paper to serve as a base between the pill and a table top and curl the paper up on the sides like a taco shell so that when the cut is made the pieces stay in the paper - as they will surely propel from the pressure once the cut is made. Plain paper is advised as anything else such as cloth or any other fibrous material will gather the pill dust or chips and they will be lost. The paper will serve as a non-porous reservoir to help you save as much medicine possible – and at the cost of these pills you'll see why you don't want even the pill dust to go to waste. Now you know why in all the movies when they show drugs being taken or sold the users' unfold pieces of paper with the drugs (usually powder) inside - they learned why and now so have you!

However you ultimately work this out, you'll need to be sure that they take the right doses each day – this will be a challenge, so start from the beginning with the goal of making it as easy and concise as possible.

Now about prescriptions; even if you have a good doctor, there are other issues in obtaining the required medicines that seem to be designed to drive a Boomer crazy. As you have probably already experienced with your own medicines, the procedure can require you to arrange a specific time for your pick-up at a pharmacy. Then you will have to stand in line and hope that when it's your turn that your medicines will not only be ready, but that the pharmacy even got word from your doctor's office to place the 'order'. In any case, be prepared for medicines not being ready, or worse, that you were told that they would be and are not.

When you go for re-fills never assume that it will happen, even if the doctor's office says it will; the pharmacy may require a faxed authorization for that refill from the doctor's office. Since your parent is not their only patient your request could take hours, and by the time they do get around to your parent's prescription it could very well be the doctor's office quitting time. You may have to wait until the next day for them to fax the prescription to the pharmacy. So to combat this you may say, "I'll just wait until my parent is 'almost' out and I'll get a re-fill ahead of time!" Not so, you cannot get refills until a date which is usually right up to the end date of the last day of the prescription. To save you time, effort and aggravation, do ask the Pharmacist for help in obtaining the paperwork from the Doctor regarding a timely refill. They already know the date of expiration and are likely to leave you a phone message just before that date. If they are not cooperative, I suggest changing to a pharmacist who will provide that level of customer service. Also ask the doctor's office about their 'policy and timing' necessary for issuing a new prescription or a continuing refill. If you are fortunate to have a doctor and pharmacy where all this can be done online consider yourself blessed.

6. DOCTORS' APPOINTMENTS

Here is another issue that seems simple enough but can end up being extremely complicated and frustrating: Doctors' office appointments.

First realize that no one likes going to the doctor and that probably goes double for your parent, so be prepared for at least a little resistance. A common sequence of events goes like this; you remind your parent of the upcoming doctor's appointment and they acknowledge the fact, but on the day of the appointment there may be some convenient lack of memory regarding the appointment. This is done in hope that the doctor's appointment will somehow go away.

Secondly, once you arrive to pick them up to take them to the doctor's office in plenty of time to make the appointment; you will find that they are no where near being ready and there will always be excuses for this and once again this is ploy number two in hopes of avoiding the appointment – it won't.

Now at this point things could become a challenge as they realize that they are losing the battle so some anger may surface. But this is not a control issue so you'll just have to remind them that you're not the bad guy, there is no bad guy, there is only "health and safety" and only for *their* benefit. Remind them that you have many of your own responsibilities to meet but are arranging time in your life to help them to stay healthy.

Another angle you must be aware of which you can avoid immediately is, "I didn't know the doctor's appointment was today!" "I thought it was next week." Here's how to stop this before it even starts; use a similar calendar, like the one for the medicines; a large one that is always in clear view, and fasten it securely to a wall or it will conveniently find its way under newspapers, the mail or anyplace that will serve as another delay, or hopefully for them a cancellation/reschedule. Writing appointments with their doctors' name and the time of day in the calendar's date square clearly removes excuses and is there as a reminder that you can have them read back to you over the phone so that each of you are aware and there can be no confusion. This is also great for any and all other important dates. Dry erase white marker boards are not advised even though they seem like a good idea. You may find that key dates and times can mysteriously be 'accidently' erased.

7. HEALTHCARE – HOMECARE – CAREGIVERS

First off, I must say that anyone in the healthcare business must be commended, for without them the world would stop.

Just as in any field there are those who are passionate and those who appear to be there just to pick up a paycheck; I have experienced both ends of this spectrum. Still, you have to know that it takes a special person to do the job they do, day in and day out. That said, if you are fortunate enough to have good experiences then consider yourself once again blessed, if not, here are a few reasons why.

If the healthcare your parent needs is in a facility then careful observation of the care of your parent and other patients will reveal a lot. Check to see how patients are treated in other rooms as you wander the halls. It may at first seem strange but most facilities can not and do not police the area and many family members and friends come to visit at all different hours, which may lead you to question the safety for all concerned. But since people are coming and going all day and into the evening you will quickly begin to recognize not only the employees, skilled nurses and the patients but the family and friends that visit as often as you do and soon you will know if you feel secure in your choice. Just be sure to remember the previous #4 on this list.

If however, you are going to employ a healthcare agency for in-home care then here are some essentials you must know.

While there are many different types of arrangements for home healthcare that involve family, friends, relatives, neighbors as well as church and social groups; I am going to focus on in-home healthcare agency/caregiver services.

The degree of healthcare your parent will require will determine the arrangement with the agency you choose. Most agencies realize that although most all situations are virtually the same that every person is unique and therefore they will always work with you to get exactly what you require; as they are in the caring business.

Those who need 24 hour around the clock care will need someone that they get along with and feel comfortable with and this may take several tryouts of individual caregivers before compatibility is met. With 24 hour care there will obviously be shifts of personnel that will have to take place at some point as even in-home caregivers that sleep at your home will need a day or two off to spend time with their families too.

If you only require a caregiver once or twice a week, that can also be arranged. But regardless of your level of healthcare needs, once a caregiver is employed you will need to be a 'Detective' of sorts to monitor your caregiver's activity.

Since you are not going to be there and the caregiver will virtually have the run of the house you will need to take these following precautions regardless of how friendly or trustworthy they initially seem.

Here are a few:

a) Lock up or remove all valuables

This means anything that is of value, within reason. You can't inventory the house all the time so "out of sight is out of mind." Even though caregivers are bonded doesn't mean that they won't have a family member or friend stop by on occasion and they are not bonded. So, to discourage any possible temptation; the removal of valuable items insures their safety.

b) Restrict 'Gift Giving'

Have a serious talk with your parent about giving items of clothing or any other items to the caregivers as a friendly gesture. Parents can sometimes get so friendly quickly with these live-in people that they tend to want to show control and generosity by gifting them with seemingly innocent items. This can escalate from a bag of items intended for Goodwill/Salvation Army to personal clothing from their closet to; dishware, radios, blankets, jewelry, furniture and well, you get the picture. Let your parent know that these people are paid to do a job and that giving them an extra

$20- or $30- once in a while to show some extra appreciation is how it should be handled. Most professionals will appreciate that; especially if there are requests of care that sometimes are above and beyond the call of duty. In some borderline cases it will keep certain caregivers 'honest'. This is an issue that you need to be the judge of, not your parent, as they are too close to the situation and emotionally involved. Also since your parent is confined to their home and their needs are met they really should have no need for cash money on hand, but if needed for the occasional emergency and for their own sense of control, it is best not to leave anything more than 20 dollars on hand for obvious reasons. Besides, you or another sibling, a friend, or even a close neighbor will undoubtedly be there every few days - so if money is absolutely needed it will be provided.

Additionally, restrict phone calls and phone usage. Whether your parent uses a cell phone or a land-line phone, restrict all phone calls for emergencies or for your parent's use. If caregivers do not have their own cell phones, that is their problem, not yours.   In any case always check your parent's monthly phone bill for unfamiliar phone calls and phone numbers. A common-sense request to the caregiver to restrict calls should be sufficient. Caregivers have children and/or parents of their own that may call or that they will need to speak with during the day or night so there will need to be some considerate allowances.

c) No visitors, boyfriends, girlfriends or children

Let the agency and the individual caregivers know that no visitors, boyfriends or children are to 'stop by'. If a caregiver needs to have her children stay for the day, tell the agency that you need a caregiver with no children. It is necessary for all involved to understand that the attention you are paying for is not to oversee someone else's children or to entertain a boyfriend or girlfriend.

On the other hand, being too strict with anyone who is caring for a loved one needs to be tempered with respect and tact - just as it is not advisable to aggravate those who prepare and serve your food – it is not wise to create an environment where there is resentment that could lead to any degree of retaliation. Just keep the relationship friendly, but on a professional level and hopefully you'll get that in return.

8. *DOCUMENT YOUR DAILY INVOLVEMENT*

At the end of what can be a physically-tiring, mentally-exhausting and emotionally-trying day, going back through each moment and chrono-logically writing down all of your responsibilities that you met will probably be the last thing you want to do – but in the end it will be to your benefit. By keeping a daily journal/account of when, where and why all things healthcare were done for your parent it will serve as an ongoing hard-copy/digital validation of your efforts for any future reference.

9. *GET ANY AGREEMENTS IN WRITING*

If you have a verbal agreement regarding any issues of healthcare for or with your parent or with other siblings regarding your daily responsibilities for your parent's healthcare issues – *get those agreements in writing and signed* by those involved!

If they refuse, then you have a problem; for no matter what you've heard, verbal agreements *are not binding!* We live in a world where state laws passed by the majority can be challenged in court. A verbal agreement means nothing.

And if your agreements are based on loving relationships and you say, "I would never ask for a signed agreement with my mother/father/sister/ brother!" all I can say is that I hope you are the exception and everything works out fine.

Senior healthcare issues can become very emotional for families – and even more so if money or inheritance is involved. So no matter how close you think you are with your parent and/or siblings or any other relatives for that matter, it is always better to be safe than sorry, so get any agreements in writing and have them signed by all parties involved.

10. KEEP ALL RECEIPTS

No matter how small or insignificant it seems at the time keep ALL receipts! They all mount up and somebody paid for them and in many cases it may have been you. Even if it was not you directly, it is very important to have a financial account as things progress. Whether your parent's rehabilitation is fortunately brief, or unfortunately long, keeping receipts provides proof of where money came from, where it went and why.

SAVE YOUR OWN LIFE!
Knowledge is power - or is it a curse?

In 2004, my 80 year old mother was diagnosed with colon cancer. After barely surviving two grueling months in the hospital for double cancer surgery (the second, to correct the first) she was able to be released. With literally only ice cubes to eat during that time, she was understandably extremely weak and unable to stand, walk or hardly move. Anticipating her release, my three siblings decided that she should go into a nursing home until she rehabilitated fully. This struck a déjà vu shockwave through me regarding the previous deadly experience with my mother-in-law. But even after I informed them of that horrible personal living nightmare experience, they still all agreed that our mother should then go into a 'nice' nursing home – they still didn't get it. I knew what the eventual outcome would be and the reasons why - and this is when my knowledge eventually became a curse.

When given the choice my mother made it clear of her preference to stay in her own home to rehabilitate as opposed to a nursing/convalescent facility if that was possible. So just prior to her release from the hospital on October 27, 2004 I entered into an agreement with a hospital-referred homecare provider for 24 hour around the clock live-in healthcare at her home.

I still had funds from my career as a designer to cover the cost for at least 3 months so that she could truly rehabilitate in her own home.

She would not be subjected to the psychotic alienating environment of a convalescent home with the constant insane and uncontrollable wailings of, "I want to die!" and far worse, from nursing home roommates. Since the three siblings did not want to contribute financially, they were not in any position to push the issue any further.

This was something that I was fortunate to be in the financial position to do. As the oldest sibling I felt it my duty to my hero Father, my cherished Grandmother and to my Grandfather that I never knew - all whom had passed on - to do this for them; to save my mother from certain death via a long and degrading physical and mental loss of life in a nursing home. I knew that they would approve and appreciate my intentions and positive actions for their wife and daughter's health and future. And I certainly could not let the experience I learned from my mother-in-law's horrific ordeal be neither forgotten, ignored nor dishonored and therefore I did what I knew was best.

Since I was able to afford temporary 24 hour care for my mother I knew that she would have a real chance to rehabilitate - in her own home - which, through my decisions *she eventually did!*

I have two younger sisters and one younger brother. These siblings did very well financially; but no offers of any financial help ever came from any of them.

My brother and his wife have no children, both have career jobs, new cars and own their own home and are approximately 20 minutes away from our mother's house.   He visited her on an average of once every 2 months, at best, and could not be counted on for anything as he was, and always has been, highly unreliable. He couldn't/

wouldn't make the effort even when requested by his own mother even though by his own words, he *"lived only minutes away."*

My youngest sister and her husband and two young girls are well off; they own new cars and a mansion with a pool on land in wine country. They live approximately 1 ½ to 2 hours away and she would make approximately 3 trips a month.

My younger sister and her husband are career teachers and are understandably not in a financial position to contribute. They live approximately 6 hours away and she would visit when she could, maybe two or three times a year at the very most, usually on holidays.

They all seemed concerned at the beginning, ready to help out physically, but not financially. But the physical help was non-existent. Once my younger sister went back home and my brother returned to his routine, the only help I received was from my youngest sister, and as I will explain later, her involvement became less and less over time.

From the moment that the 24 hour cancer rehabilitation healthcare began I made trips to and from my mother's home 3 to 4 times each week. The 2 hour 68 mile round trip required about 5 to 10 additional miles in the form of local errands and not-so-local trips to her doctors.

I make all of these comparisons to point out that anyone who decides to take on this responsibility will soon realize that initial concerns and involvement by family fade fast and therefore it becomes a solitary as well as all-consuming continual task. There was always something to do and payment required.

In my case, on the days that I did not need to make the trip, I instead spent considerable time on the phone with specific and peripheral agencies regarding her health and safety issues. I arranged for a wheelchair and portable toilet through Medical and personally provided her with a bathtub chair, a walker, blood pressure testing apparatus, a new washing machine and numerous other material needs. And there was always ongoing associated healthcare and personal paperwork to process. This was only the beginning of a sacrificed lifestyle for me, my wife and son as I was literally 'on call' on a daily basis.

My mother had several regular doctors and several specialists whose scheduled appointments between them guaranteed near weekly visits. In order to take her to her doctor's appointments I would carry her down her home's very short set of stairs, set her into my car and put the wheel chair in back. After the appointments I would utilize the time at her house wisely by tending to her other household needs. I also walked her dog around the neighborhood while she was in the hospital and continued to do so several times a week once she returned. Then I'd do her grocery shopping, as well as pick up her medicines; which could often be a frustrating and time-consuming effort. *See Baby Boomer Checklist Section: Medicine Prescriptions and Dosages.*

Dealing with live-in home health caregivers was a new world for me in which the reality was that some healthcare workers take advantage - which was the case with some caregivers employed by the initial homecare provider company. I now had to monitor the caregivers' phone use, suspected food stealing, clothes stealing, and unauthorized visits of the care-givers' friends and other issues that went on when I was not there. Responsible agencies/caregivers can be an issue.

  Each and every trip to her house would end up consuming the entire day with departures from my home usually anywhere from 8 to 11 AM and then return trips wherein I usually left late in the evening, many times as late as 12 midnight. I would arrive at my home exhausted and on occasion I would fall asleep in my car in my own driveway. These trips took a toll on my 16 year old car resulting in at least four different break-downs due to the wear incurred by the frequent long-distance round trips. Although this became an emotional as well as physical job; I chose out of love for my mother and the undying love for my dear grandmother and father to keep up the pace and the personal cost.

  Once she was able to become ambulatory enough to use a walker and get into a car, my youngest sister would *occasionally* relieve me of some of the responsibility, mainly in regard to a doctors' appointment, this however took place months later and was rare. Also as I would tend to stay all day and late into the evening; on the few days a month she could make the trip she would come late and leave early; granted she lived further away, but it still limited her time and therefore her help.

I soon realized that if ever in the future my mother needed financial help due to the return of cancer or any other convalescing situation that it would definitely not come from my siblings. And if ever that time came, I might not be in the same financial position to cover her costs either. So I investigated a term that was completely new to me; Reverse Mortgage.

The house my parents purchased back in the 1950s had long since been paid off and my mother now owned a house of considerable value. If needed in the future, the reverse mortgage would supply the funds required to cover her healthcare based on her past 24 hour care situation. The only alternate financial suggestion to a reverse mortgage, which came from my youngest sister's husband, would not cover the average total monthly amount - only barely half - so who would cover the monthly balance if and when needed? Realizing no financial help would be coming from my siblings, ever, nor possibly from me depending on future finances; to protect herself my mother decided to apply for the reverse mortgage.

Prior to her bout with cancer, my mother had left her purse on a bus; it was never retrieved. She lost her California ID, her Social Security card, Medicare card and all other forms of important personal identification that she kept in her purse. These crucial personal identifications needed to be replaced before we could begin the reverse mortgage process. Since each ID item was dependent upon the other, it became a conundrum of frustration for her and me and a highly time-consuming effort as well.

This whole ordeal involved written letters, verifications, copies, faxes, phone calls and long waits for return mail with forms to fill-out and then more waiting and more follow-up phone calls. Unfortunately, *at that time* hard copies via mail and faxes were required as there was virtually no processing done through the internet. I see that now Social Security promotes the use of their online services; possibly other agencies have followed suit.

While her birth certificate was not lost with her purse, it was lost in her house and could not be located. That became another issue that required my time and attention to have a new one verified, reproduced and then sent by mail.

So I now began a secondary job of obtaining these IDs which became as time-consuming as her health and safety care issues. This new process literally took months, plus in the wake of 911 the security measures regarding personal identity were severely increased. I felt it; not only in obtaining the IDs but with the duration of time needed to process all paperwork needed by the mortgage company. The agents I worked with said that the process should normally have taken 2, maybe 3 months maximum - but instead it took nearly 6 months before the procedure was completely finalized.

Meanwhile all continued doctors' appointments and co-pays, medicine pick-ups and co-pays, grocery purchases, drug store item purchases and taking her dog to the veterinarian and paying for his medicine and visits, gas costs for my car's round-trips, as well as the physical duties that needed to be done around her house, all remained my sole responsibilities   Once again, I was fortunate to be in the position to take on this responsibility, but it began to come with a personal cost. This personal cost was that it left me absolutely no time to spend with my own family or to maintain my career.

As a successful independent artist and designer I had an extremely deadline-intense workload over the past decade. The independent nature of my career *initially* allowed me the flexible schedule to perform all these many jobs for my mother.   The fact that all of my career projects centered on meeting extremely tight deadlines made it impossible to seek or accept any jobs during the years I cared for my mother; so my career was put on hold.

Care for a parent comes with sacrifices, for everyone, including extended family. The husband, wife, son, daughter, boyfriend, girlfriend or partner of a Boomer will also be affected. So for those moments that will test your stress levels; take a breath and remember your goals of health and safety. Healthcare for a parent is not a 40 hour a week job with weekends off; it's virtually a 24 hour a day job, 7 days a week. Because even if not physically-involved for all of the 7 days a week; you are mentally on the job, all the time.

At the end of 6 tedious months I finally had her entire personal ID profile intact and could begin the reverse mortgage process. We discussed the situation at length and to make a difficult process easier we agreed that I would acquire the Legal General Power of Attorney (with Durable Provision) plus the Legal Durable Power of Attorney for Healthcare. She declined the option to have a secondary Power Of Attorney added.

The whole idea of the benefits of a reverse mortgage was to insure that she would have the funds to cover her healthcare in the event of any future health-related issues.

I contacted a mortgage company in a town nearby my home and began the process early in 2004. By law, all mortgage companies must send an evaluator out to any senior who is applying for a reverse mortgage to personally discuss the process. Additionally the senior is required to take a test so that they are clear and aware of the procedure and its purpose. She was in full lucid control of her faculties and passed this verbal and written test.

From the beginning of the reverse mortgage process, my mother and I discussed and agreed that I would need to eventually be reimbursed for any monies I contributed to keep her in her own home as opposed to the negative downward spiral of a 'nursing home'. Under the circumstances this was justifiably fair; she fully understood, agreed and thanked me on many occasions for all I had done and was still doing. In addition, in order to keep maintaining her living conditions, I needed to maintain mine. Even with my initial funds replaced I could not continue to devote the time needed to keep her alive without receiving some sort of income. This would be impossible for anyone unless they were independently wealthy. I would either have to quit her ongoing health and safety maintenance, or continue. And just like any of the other siblings with career jobs, if they were to take my place and therefore quit their jobs, *they too* would have needed some sort of monetary supplement to stay alive. So my mother agreed that in order to keep her alive she would temporarily help keep me alive by providing a bare minimum monthly amount to live on. *This survival level of income was only temporary, as we agreed, until she no longer needed the level of attention and oversight I was providing.* This became a verbal agreement between a mother and her first born son that I never once thought to get in writing. Trusting in that verbal agreement would turn out to be a huge, monumental mistake on my part. And one that you, Parent or Boomer, no matter what kind of a loving trusting relationship you have with your mother or father, son or daughter, sister or brother will find that under certain circumstances your agreement can not only be ignored but can be turned against you.

Even though on many distinct occasions my mother had expressed her sincere thanks for my sacrifice and assistance regarding her care and was fully aware of her agreement with me regarding my survival-level allowance; I could have never ever imagined the eventual horrific outcome.

During the 6 months of the reverse mortgage process there were many pre-requisite issues to be completed at my mother's house. So, through on-site meetings and phone conversations I arranged and oversaw the initiation and completion of the termite inspection, small but important household repairs, roofing issues and repairs, the tearing-up and re-paving of an entirely new driveway, as well as the tear-down, reinforcement and replacement of a property-line concrete wall. In most cases each of these projects required my on-site presence.

The three siblings stayed completely uninvolved and to this day have no knowledge as to the deep involvement required by me in this matter, nor the health matters, nor the homecare matters, nor any of the other matters. I now realize that keeping them informed would have been smart and to my advantage but at the time it seemed ridiculous to file a daily report to people who obviously didn't care – whereas I should have been doing it all along for my own benefit.

Even as she gradually got better while still under live-in healthcare supervision the lack of control in her life began to show in the rebellion of doctors' instructions and orders. This show of 'frustration/ rebellion' is natural, I saw it with my mother-in-law, sometimes the only control they have is to say "No", but it is equally frustrating and anti-productive for those devoted to seeing that their loved ones get better.

After a while her attitude changed from one who was appreciative of the concerned help given; to one who now expected it. Although this also became very frustrating for me, I understood and continued my daily responsibilities but had to remind her that all of this, everything, even that which seemed bad, was for *her health and safety,* this wasn't a control issue, this was all about her health and safety!   That was my bottom-line mantra and goal; "Health and Safety".

Eventually, all of the reverse mortgage requirements were met and the electronic deposit was made in a local reputable regional bank. A non-checking account was created as per the process that she and I shared at her request. Even though to have any siblings on the account was unnecessary as they were all uninvolved, I did make the offer to my youngest sister - but she declined. I was aware that it would be prudent to find an investment for her funds, but it was not a priority as I was still busy with her daily issues of health and safety. So I reserved any decisions until I gathered more information. The three siblings were aware of the reverse mortgage funds; however, they offered no other viable investment suggestions.

An experience I had well over a decade ago, whereby I was unable to withdraw my personal funds from my own bank due to a major electrical outage in my area motivated me to take matters into my own hands in regard to banking.

I preferred to withdraw cash and then deposit only when needed to pay bills. This was my personal normal procedure for well over a decade *prior* to the healthcare issues with my mother. It was/is a smart safety precaution while living in Southern California when the potential 'Big One' could knock out electricity for days or weeks.

As a side note, for a very helpful but truly scary video, especially for Californians, watch the Los Angeles Fire Department video on Earthquake Preparedness. The part about how cash/banking distribution will be handled in the case of an extended electrical outage sounds like an apocalyptic sci-fi horror story. This will be of interest to citizens of any city where a potential catastrophic event could cripple normal everyday life functions. Therefore, my personal policy toward 'banking' continues to make sense.

As my mother improved, the amount of my responsibilities did not lessen; now all the projects that were not previous priorities came to the forefront and were addressed. For many years she rented a spare room to local university and college students. For quite some time after her last renter left, her back bedroom and bathroom were literally closed-off to the rest of the house due to the black mold that grew out of control in both of those rooms. The three siblings were completely aware of this ugly mess for many months but no help was offered to do anything about it. So I, with a history of asthma, cut up the wall-to-wall carpet backed by black mold and disposed of it.

When she was able to walk and gradually resume her daily routine, I set her up with Meals on Wheels so she could have warm food delivered. I also registered and arranged for her to have use of CityRide, a local minimal-fee taxi service for seniors. She could now make short trips to the local drugstore, market, department store, and so on. The benefits of these short trips were priceless as they contributed toward her regaining her sense of freedom and independence.

Meanwhile, my youngest sister asked her older sister to relieve her of the delivered grocery market orders since she could do that from where she lived via the phone or internet. To my knowledge this has been my younger sister's sole contribution.

My mother's primary doctor, while a great guy, had an incredibly frustrating phone staff that would put you on hold – and never come back. This eventually brought my youngest sister to tears to the point that she wouldn't even deal with scheduling her mother's appointments anymore. So to cure this situation I began to drop by his office in person on my way to her house to confirm appointments and insure that I was able to talk with him personally regarding her medical issues.

My mother eventually successfully regained her health and independence from rehabilitating in her own home to the point where she only needed health-care several days a week.

This accomplishment was of great satisfaction for both of us to have reached the goal of recovery to near normal health status prior to cancer.

Now I could end my financial and healthcare arrangement with her and resume my career to earn the level of income I and my family had worked hard over the years to achieve and maintain.

But unfortunately, this was not to be.

One early evening after a doctor's appointment and dinner at a local favorite restaurant of ours we arrived at her home. As I was unlocking the front door she had just reached the top step of her short set of stairs. She descended and ascended these stairs countless times when I was not there, but this time she slipped and twisted backwards while still holding onto the stair's railing. This sudden twist broke her upper femur.

I carried her inside and called for an ambulance which soon arrived and took her to the emergency room of her local hospital.

The question of why had I not been assisting her up the stairs is a question that can bring up the possibility of guilt feelings. If anything similar happens to you, please avoid this trap – it is not your fault. Here is a perfect example: on any given day before leaving my mother's house if time allowed I would sometimes walk her down the block and back. Although she didn't need assistance, one time I held her hand all the way to within several houses of hers and I let go to step up on the grass off the sidewalk. A few steps later she got distracted by a bird in a tree and fell. The fall was a gentle one on soft grass and she was alright. The moral is that unless you literally hold their hand 24 hours a day you cannot insure that they receive no harm. The behavior of any other person is beyond your control. You cannot be held guilty for not being at the right place at the right time. What about all of the times when you're not there?

When she was finally able to come home from the hospital after a pinned-bone operation; the three siblings once again attempted to lobby for her to go into a convalescent/nursing home. *It now became all too apparent that their loyalties were to their shares of inheritance money through the sale of her home once she vacated it, never to return - not what was best for their mother.*

I entered into a new agreement with a different in-home healthcare service, which proved to be a much better arrangement.

This latest broken femur ordeal was a far worse rehabilitation effort than the cancer ordeal due to the fact that with cancer she just needed to get her strength back, with the broken femur she had to endure the frustration of 'learning' to walk again.

This frustration turned into rebellion as the scheduled in-home physical therapist's requests regarding leg exercises were ignored or done with token efforts. This proved very frustrating and counter-productive toward the whole point of home rehabilitation. Even with a history of blood circulation issues, she had already been lax on the elevation of her feet as per her doctor's orders prior to this breakage incident. She administered her own glaucoma drops incorrectly and when instructed properly; continued incorrectly. Medicine, of which there were three to six different types to take throughout the day, were also conveniently forgotten from time to time and strict enforcement by caregivers became imperative. These deliberately rebellious actions were certainly due to the frustration of her learning-to-walk-again issue as she loved to go for long walks. She was actually very well known locally due to her regular long-walk excursions over the decades.

To help ease her emotional transitional condition I positioned a portable toilet right next to her bed that required no walking to use. And by her use of a walker to get around her home her health care was reduced from 24 hours a day to approximately 12 hours a day. Caregivers would arrive each morning and leave each night. So she was on her own for a couple hours before going to bed at night and a couple hours in the morning after waking.

As the months went by she once again improved to her previous health levels by rehabilitating in her own home. This was a reality that would not have been if she were in a convalescent home!

In early August 2007, upon arriving at my mother's house for an extremely important cardiologist appointment I was ambushed by my youngest sister and accused of stealing my mother's money - not questioned, accused.

And once again it was 'money trumps health' as my sister had somehow poisoned or convinced our mother to cancel this very important cardiologist appointment in order to stage this ambush based on ignorance.

I was completely shocked and dismayed, but before I could say anything amid the accusations, my youngest sister threatened 'legal' action while she held out her phone for whoever was on the other end to hear any statements I made. I looked at my mother who amazingly also had an air of anger about her and it was at that moment that I had no choice but to leave.

After being submerged in a flood of emotions as I drove away, I finally surfaced back to reality to realize that I had sacrificed my life, my own family's standard of living, as well as my career and my time – and apparently for nothing. Well, that's not true, although that's how it felt, actually my efforts saved her life *twice* so it was worth it, The fact that the siblings *and my mother* reduced my whole considerate, dedicated, nearly 4 year effort down to nothing more than a 'money issue' was sad and shocking.

NO GOOD DEED GOES UNPUNISHED!
True Life Present Day Cautionary Story #2

How much money is a life worth? Priceless; isn't that what all of us Boomers were raised to believe - and know to be true?

Approximately 10 months after the ambush and the accusations and with no contact with any other 'family members', I was contacted by an L.A.P.D. detective who wanted to talk with me regarding 'stolen money' of an elder. Unbelievable as it was at the time, my youngest sister had literally called the cops with these totally false accusations. Since I had nothing to hide I let my self-righteousness override my common sense and met with the two detectives without a lawyer present. Although thoroughly stupid on my part (without legal representation) we agreed on a date that I would hand in copies of all the receipts that I had saved that *accounted for all of the allegedly 'stolen money'*.

BUT - on the Saturday morning *FOUR DAYS BEFORE* the agreed upon officially-scheduled Tuesday report date for me to hand-in those receipts to the detective – I was arrested!!

On that Saturday morning my wife and I were abruptly woken to the hard rapid pounding on our front door accompanied by loud shouting by the L.A.P.D.!

In Los Angeles it is commonly known that you and your family could easily become shooting victims by these 'officers of the law' in such a circumstance. Thus being jolted awake from my sleep, I feared the worst and yelled to them through the front door to meet me on the back deck of the house. As I went out onto the back deck, *five* police officers with their loaded guns drawn and pointed straight at me, began their macho yelling routine and accused me of trying to avoid arrest – I live backed by the Santa Monica Mountains and their slopes end in my backyard – there is literally no where to go. Our neighbors, whose two-story house allowed them a perfect view of the whole scene taking place on my back deck, told me that they would attest as witnesses to the fact that I was not trying to escape anything or anyone. My 'back deck' actions were to insure that my family, including animal family members, would remain as safe as possible – and I succeeded.

The Los Angeles Police Department has earned their internationally-known, fully-justified and documented reputation for wide-spread police brutality and killing of innocents for good reason.

Due to the blatant outright lie and set-up by the L.A.P.D. 'Detective' I was denied my right to submit my receipts *on the agreed-upon date* and therefore could now only do so in a trial. This was only the beginning of the systematic deceit, lies and manipulation of the (In)Justice System that I was to experience. And as I found myself arrested, in handcuffs and then in Los Angeles County jail awaiting arraignment; the quote, "No good deed goes unpunished" became a horrible unjust truth.

I have lived my life of 59 years on this planet as an honest, non-materialistic person with a spotlessly clean record. I am an artist; I am certainly not a criminal, and I received no monetary gain from this ordeal.

Here is a truly sad but truly life-saving fact that you can learn from my experience - *money can trump everything* - friends and even family relationships dissolve when money is at stake. Unfortunately, this isn't cynicism, it's the truth.

However, *had* I originally agreed with my siblings to put our mother in a convalescent home to rehabilitate from her 2 cancer surgeries, by now she would no longer be with us and I would have received at least one-quarter of the sale of her home as stipulated in her Will. But instead, she is safe, alive and living in her own home. For all of my efforts the result is that I am now penniless, in debt, with a felony conviction, 200 hours of community service, on 5 years formal probation (which will surely be extended by request from the D.A.) *and with a restitution payment that totals <u>all</u> of her bills, healthcare expenses, in-home 24 hour care expenses and <u>all</u> other expenses!*
In other words *I have to pay <u>ALL</u> the money – everything that was spent to keep her alive and healthy in her own home for nearly a four year period!* An absolutely insane outcome!

Why Did I Not Fight This In Court?

Initially, before I was given a public defender and then fortunate enough to eventually retain an attorney, I had planned to go to trial. But what I learned quickly about a juried trial through my own limited but intense encounter with the 'justice' system and through my attorney was that it is never wise to put your fate in the hands of 12 people if you have the option to make your own decision.

What I have learned would be worthy of a small tome on the subject, but instead I will list the reasons pertinent to my situation and you can extend them on to any other situation and see why our current 'justice' system is nothing more than a processing machine of injustice.

The following is a complete and utter deadly joke that dispels all that you thought you knew, were told or have been raised to believe - whether through school, your parents, news, movies, books and TV. Specifically; *"You have the right to remain silent. Anything you say can and will be used against you in a court of law. You have the right to have an attorney present during questioning. If you cannot afford an attorney, one will be appointed for you.*" Everyone is aware of this basic constitutional right, we've heard it our whole lives, but I was blatantly denied this right of legal representation even though I was deemed indigent by the court and therefore could not afford an attorney and therefore one should have been appointed to me. But, unlike in the movies, no one would step forward and challenge this injustice that I was being dealt. Any public or private attorney who would take my case would immediately be considered a non-processing and judge-challenging troublemaker. This pedestrian processing and denial of basic constitutional rights issue continues because most all attorneys, public and private, repeatedly end up before the same judges, case after case, therefore the attorney/judge relationship is based on 'not rocking the boat', even in the slightest.

A newly-hired attorney from the firm that initially represented me at my sentencing was representing me pro bono the day it all went down. The judge's decision (which was made in consort with the D.A. *and* the Deputy Public Defender) after viewing my financial evaluation for restitution was to uphold the previous per month amount even though the court knew I was indigent. My attorney argued that my current indigent status was not being considered - the judge said, "He can scrimp". I was also denied my basic constitutional rights of legal representation going forward! It was made clear that I could not have a public defender. When my attorney questioned this, she was shut down. As we left the courtroom she was so stunned that when I asked her for advice she was speechless. When I questioned her again she said she had never encountered this blatant disregard for anyone's rights and made it clear she was off my case - and in her bewilderment she had no advice as to whom I should seek for justice.

Remember: *All courtroom dramas are pure fantasy.*

With that said: here are 4 good reasons why I didn't fight this in court.

1. Lies.

Lies by the people 'involved'; lies by the L.A.P.D. Detective; lies by the Judge; lies by the D.A.; lies by my own Public Defender and lies by the alleged 'Victim" – whose life I literally saved twice by my actions and concern. There is only one victim and it is not her.

My ongoing 'justice' system experience only confirmed my previous understanding and belief of the use of lies with devious unjust intent for self-interest coupled with soulless 'legal' abuse and manipulation that results in a total lack of humanity and true justice.

I was told recently by a highly reputable source that a retired, high ranking L.A.P.D. officer was once asked "How do you know if a law officer is lying?" his response was, "Were his lips moving?" I rest my case.

2. *Peers.*

Based on the above and the fact that no jury is truly made up of your 'peers' makes this a battle you can't win from the start. Peers? In my opinion the concept is nearly impossible to achieve when you really think about it. A jury would have to consist of 12 people who have had the same experiences as you – not only in life, but specifically in regard to this situation, for example; watching their mother-in-law die in a convalescent home after going in for a broken hip - and therefore understanding the reasoning for a 'peer's' actions. They would also have to be people who were self-employed, who made considerable money and were used to handling such and therefore knew the difference between money, which can always be made again, and the priceless value of a life, that cannot be made again. Additionally, they would have the same moral beliefs, know the difference between right and wrong, have the ability to use 'common-sense' and have the intelligence to see through lies and discern the truth.   Plus if they *did* have any of the same experiences - they would be excluded (?!). Peers: A farce and a totally unachievable concept.

3. *Cost of an attorney.*

   With the cut-backs and horror stories of the overload of cases Public Defenders' have, I knew that I needed to speak to someone who was not based in the Criminal Injustice Building. (See #4). Not only is, "No good deed goes unpunished" a true quote but; "It's times like this when you find out who your real friends are" is another. My brother-in-law is my real brother; he knew who I was and who I am. If not for his own innate ability to recognize another human being for whom they are, but for the insight and understanding of seeing the way that I treated his own mother. He literally saved my life by lending me the money to hire a real attorney.

A paid attorney will spend time with you, because you pay him/her for their services, unlike public defenders who generally have literally dozens of cases and can never truly handle your case to any degree that the life-in-the-balance situation of the threat of prison brings.

Bottom-line is that my attorney said I would probably win the case *but* I would end up paying him nearly the same amount or a very large portion of what I was being accused of 'stealing'. And worse, if I didn't win, for whatever reason, I would go straight to prison to serve out a sentence of 4 to 6 years.

So you can see why coupled with the previous #1 and #2 above to enter a plea bargain is the only sure way to stay out of prison. Since knowing this, I would never ever trust in 12 people to decide my fate if I had the choice, and thankfully I had that choice.

Admitting to "No Contest" (Nolo Contendere) means that you will not 'contest" the verdict and therefore you will give up all your rights to question any 'witnesses' or 'evidence' or to have a 'deliberation'. In actuality it means that you are not admitting to the guilt but have 'no way' of 'contesting' the accusation - in my case I did not have the unlimited financial resources to win a court trial – *which as we are all well aware of by now is what truly dictates 'justice'.*

During the plea bargaining phase my attorney told me that not only were my siblings going to state that they spent more time with our mother than I did but so did their spouses! Unbelievable! When he told me this I realized the depth and quantity of outright lies that these people were willing to state as truth. I was also fully enlightened as to whom I was dealing with; the truly soulless who apparently had no consciences.

4. *Cost of a Public Defender.*

An even higher cost, one that doesn't involve money, comes with this choice. The Public Defender who was eventually assigned to me became another horrific experience on top of the accusation, the arrest and the experience in L.A. County Jail. She had the most incredibly negative attitude imaginable; she was curt, unpleasant and had a single Chatty Cathy pull-string response to everything I asked or said, which was; "You're going to jail." Wow! And she was to represent me, in my defense?

I wasn't aware that the statistical reality of court case loads is that only a single digit percentage of cases actually go to trial. So she was just trying to intimidate me into a plea bargain to make her life easier since I told her initially that I wanted a trial. That all changed later, when I found out through my paid attorney what I was really up against. Still, I thought that a sliver of compassion and a moment of intelligent unbiased exchange of dialogue between the public defender and me should have been appropriate, necessary and required - but no, that was not the case. I was appalled. But wait it gets better. My first time in court with her she was late, almost got into an argument with the judge, did get into an argument with the court clerk, and left the courtroom telling me that the clerk was a "bitch" and that another public defender would handle my case today! The other P.D. didn't have a clue regarding me or my case and just asked for another court date. After that I realized that I could not go forward with this unprofessional negative person; if I stayed with her I was dead before I started. Then I realized that I was just one of countless others whose lives are in the hands of public defenders like her - a sad, very sad situation of alienation and bare minimum representation. Most public defenders don't even know the particulars of the 'accused' person's case until they are actually in court for the first time with them and then they usually ask for a continuance so that they can make time to actually review the case. This situation will then send the defendant back to jail if they were unable to secure bail and even more time of having your life put on hold waiting to have just a few words with the public defender assigned to you.   This was painfully evident when weeks went by and just prior to the pre-trial hearing court date from out of nowhere the public defender called me to see if I had anything else to contribute as evidence ... wait, what? No contact whatsoever for literally weeks and then just days before this very important court date she contacts me! When I informed her that I had an attorney (thanks to the compassion and concern of my Brother-In-Law) she said she was going to appear in court anyway – she didn't.

The only person throughout this whole ordeal that was on the side of fairness and justice was the Judge who determined my bail at the arraignment. His apparent insight was that this was obviously a family matter gone horribly wrong and by review-ing my spotless record and age he verified this assumption by lowering my bail down to *one-sixth* of the original request by the D.A. My attorney stated that this fact alone would weigh heavily in my favor if I went to trial, but I realized that the only sure way to avoid the threat of prison was to decline a trial and to enter into a plea bargain; which is what I did. A plea bargain usually consists of an admission of guilt in exchange for a lighter sentence. *This false admission amounts to nothing less than legal-blackmail.* Innocent defendants without funds for serious legal representation are shamefully manipulated into guilty pleas by this unjust ploy every day across America.

Motivations?

It's natural that in many families, one may find certain degrees of love, hate and jealousy that siblings harbor between each other and toward the first born. In my case I was fortunate to have spent wonderful quality time with our father and grandmother, unfortunately for the siblings they did not. After living and growing up with them for much of my youth and teens, once I moved out I was ready for a new world of relationships. Our considerable age difference was a natural contribution toward our distant relationships and we never really had that much in common, so except for the occasional holiday we did not maintain contact. My own life with my family, my dedicated 24/7/365 work schedule, focus on my art career and my own personal interests happily and thankfully took up every aspect of my life. So, it's quite possible that their misinterpretations and assumptions about our distant relationships contributed to already existing deep-seated feelings of jealousy and resentment directed toward their older brother for being born first and having a life - or not, I'll never really know.

Regarding my youngest sister's obsessive motives; even though she was the only one who definitely knew what I was responsible for on a daily/weekly/monthly basis regarding our mother's health and safety, she still persisted in this attack. Her actions and vindictive false accusations were, and still are, unconscionable.

When our father died she was very young and therefore was literally raised without a father; which can create abandonment issues. (I have personal experience with this condition as my wife's father passed away when she was very young and for her it was the same as if he had 'left her' and sometimes for women especially, that can have profound repercussions of abandonment issues later in life.) My youngest sister also married a fireman, a man with a profession that keeps him away from the house for days and nights; he is literally an absent husband/father. This is a classic example of abandonment fallout as she was drawn to what she knew, in this case a male/father figure who is not around.

For the time that she and I communicated during the years of our mother's condition, which was mostly on the phone, we became somewhat close. I believe that she took this false 'embezzlement' claim personally and her rage stems from a very strange phone message after the fact of, "I thought you loved me." This statement shows more concern for her feelings than for our mother's well-being and seemed too unbalanced a statement for me to offer a response.

After the initial ambush and accusations I avoided and ignored her completely, which was possibly to my own detriment as it only intensified her ego-driven rage.

Additionally, I've been informed that her oldest daughter has recently enrolled as a state university student; this requires a considerable tuition that she may have been counting on from her share of their inheritance.

Since she cannot count on her twin brother or her older sister; she now has to carry the sole responsibility of the 'health and safety' of her mother that I successfully maintained for nearly four years. She will soon find out, if she hasn't already, that her 'victory' will have a major impact of inconvenience on her previously charmed life-style.

True Facts

So, to sum up this horrendous experience, which continues every day with the threat of having my freedom taken away until full 'restitution' is paid, here are the true facts.

1) Ironically, *I actually saved my mother money*; approximately $25,000.00 per year verses the amount, as a home-owner, she would have paid otherwise.

2) Statistics show that women over 80 *rarely* rehabilitate in nursing/convalescent homes to the point of returning to their own home/life-style. As the legal profession refers to it; convalescent homes are where "people go to die".

3) Even in the highly unlikely possibility that she had survived the first rehabilitation in a convalescent home; the second one for her broken femur would never have resulted in a successful rehabilitation because it would have required concentrated effort and therapy that these facilities' can not and do not provide.

The completely distracting hospital ward environment makes it nearly impossible for a parent/patient to concentrate and coupled with physical therapies that are not practiced daily, but only once or twice a week at best, the patient's disoriented mind loses concentration of the goal.

4) Money was never an issue – it was a tool, a tool for her survival - I certainly gained no profit.

5) My mother and I had an agreement for the re-imbursement of my personal out-of-pocket funds from her initial home-rehabilitation from cancer and funds so that I could maintain the minimum survival level needed to insure that she survived and rehabilitated within her own home and secure environment. She knew this as I reminded her of our agreement regularly and she was pleased to be able to help me, help her (I will never really know

whether her negative reaction was due to Alzheimer's, or the mental poisoning from my youngest sister, or that she truly forgot. Possibly even her concern over the value of money over the value of her own health and safety had become more important due to her changing mental state.) 6) Had my mother not incurred the broken femur, the agreement we had would have terminated - but because of this second consequential incident the agreement continued which is why the funds continued to be used. This was the reason for the reverse mortgage safety net in the first place.

7) The fact that the siblings interpreted this as some way for me to 'steal' money is ludicrous. The irony is that I could have furthered my career and easily made up to four times the amount of my agreement with my mother had I continued with my design career and agreed with the siblings to admit her to a nursing facility.

8) Caring for, and being responsible for another human being is not an easy job and while it does offer the satisfaction of helping another human when they need it the most, it can also literally deprive you of your own life. Anyone who has had

a child already knows this. The sacrifice made by myself and my family impacted our lifestyle in a devastating negative ripple-effect that we are still feeling and will continue to feel for years to come. 9) *The decision I made has kept her alive, healthy, rehabilitated and in her own home. It was a success and I will always know that its' worth was priceless.*

Parent Boomer Relationships

I must set the record straight and divulge some-thing I have not yet mentioned and that is that I never really had a 'good' relationship with my mother. Other than our mutual interest in movies and music, we never saw eye to eye on anything.

This is not uncommon to a certain extent between any parent and child of any generation and certainly not to us Boomers who experienced and embraced nothing less than a revolutionary cultural change from the traditional values, ideas and beliefs of our parents. This separation of beliefs had an immense impact and created the historic "Generation Gap".

My mother contributed to this dynamic by possessing a sweet surface with an underlying condescending negative nature. This attitude coupled with her lack of interaction with me as a child could have been an issue, but since I was an imaginative budding artist the time spent alone as a child was never an issue as I rather preferred it. Interestingly though, in the months after her cancer ordeal in some rare honest moments the siblings each voiced their own unprovoked realizations that she was never really that warm or interactive with them either. It is times like these when peoples' true feelings and insights surface.

I've come to realize now that her level of affection was based on her attitude and personality and that she probably never had the ability to express or feel true compassionate emotions, or if she did, they always seemed to be masked by superficiality.

On any given day she would test the limits of our diametrically-opposed views by inevitably initiating some sort of argument, in person or on the phone. I eventually avoided contact with her for many of her younger, healthier years due to the constant negative attitude she upheld. This was not a psychological maternal issue of avoidance, this was a wise decision, as I could no longer debate issues with someone who couldn't be bothered to inform herself on the ideas she supposedly stood for. It became ridiculous, tiring and a pure waste of time and energy. It's strange how some people feel the need to immediately find or point out the negative *before* exploring the positive of any given situation.

Now, two things may come to mind as you read the previous paragraphs: One, "Hey that's the kind of relationship I have/had with my mother/father/ son/daughter!", or, "Well, now I understand, he just took advantage of someone he really disliked and probably felt as though he was vindicated in anything he did!" Both are valid assumptions - BUT - while getting along with any family member, relative, friend, neighbor, co-worker, business-associate, boyfriend, girlfriend, life-partner, wife or husband or anyone you are in a position to interact with on a regular basis may become trying, difficult or seemingly impossible – *it does not affect what is right and what is wrong.*

I knew what was right morally as well as academically. In this case if she went to a convalescent home it probably meant dying there – it would only be a matter of time – and I had the means and knowledge to prevent that outcome. I can live at peace with this decision as the alternative of knowing and then not acting would have been mournfully regretful.

My Grandmother and my Father were both positive, intelligent, loving role-model influences in my life. My love and concern for them is what I know to be the motivation for the manifested actions made by me on their behalf for her child and his wife. And certainly the traditional Boomer-imprinted 'duty of the first born son' contributed to my motivation to take charge in this situation from the very beginning; to do the right thing for my mother's health and safety.

A really ironic sad outcome from this whole ordeal was that in the time I spent with my mother we actually seemed to get along much better. We were enjoying each other's company and even went to a few movies, drove around to look at

Christmas lights, went to see James Van Praagh, went to the opera, cruised LAX to see the trippy Light Portal and even had some decent conversations. We were in the process of building a better relationship. And then to have it all torn down – the good feelings from the success of the physical health issues, as well as from the closer relationship we were developing together – was/is tragic.

Common Sense

Now for the most telling part; had any of the siblings done what I did they would have had to quit their jobs also. If anyone of them stopped to consider this fact the obvious would remain. This is why I had to have an agreement with my mother - to maintain my survival so that I could maintain hers. My agreement was with her, not between other members of the family. I do not know of their personal agreements with her or with anyone else - it is not my business. They made it their business *to stay uninvolved* regarding our mother's condition and I certainly did not receive concerned requests from them daily, weekly or monthly about those issues either; *only when they felt that their 'inheritance' was being 'spent' did they get 'involved'* - which speaks volumes.

And if my actions were seen by them as a total money issue, then why not just remove me from our mother's Will? While still totally unjust, this common-sense handling of the situation on their part would have achieved the same financial end. My 'share', that which kept our mother alive, rehabilitated and in her home, could have been applied to the falsely-accused 'stolen' amount and they would still get their 'justified' share. But obviously that was not enough for them, as some very ugly hidden anger and resentment surfaced with an agenda to fulfill that this situation served as a catalyst to complete. Their need and desire to see severe punishment and suffering dealt to me and my family was and still is apparent. If I've since been removed from the 'Will' - their three-way split will greatly benefit them with the added full 'restitution' amount that I have to pay to them. Yes, to them, because if not paid off when our mother dies, payment continues to *them*.

EPILOGUE

My only parent/boomer convalescent home situation/experience prior to that of my mother-in-law was with my Grandmother. At a spry 80 years old she was a manager of a 12 unit apartment complex in a neighboring city. Born in 1900, she was one of the 'real' women that made America: strong, smart, loving and wouldn't suffer fools.

She was very healthy until one day while avoiding a bee on the front steps of a ground-floor apartment she suffered a small stroke and although she lost her balance she was able to grab a railing and fortunately didn't fall. But that 'mini-stroke' incident led to the inevitable stay in a convalescent home in a city near her daughter's home. Through the obvious disparity of seeing her in that desolate situation, my uncle and my mother arranged for her to stay at my mother's home. Fortunately, her stroke was not severe and she did not require 24 hour care. She could be left alone when her daughter went to work at her part-time job that was within walking distance of her home.

My mother experienced the caring of, and for, her mother and knew the dedication required and the physical and emotional toll it took to care for a parent. This should have served as an education when her time came to be more understanding and empathetic toward myself, her friends, neighbors, family and all others who cared about her. But the irony of this situation is that for whatever reasons, she did not benefit by her own experience and instead actually focused on petty and negative issues, rather than the issues of her own health and of the concern others had for her well-being.

This leads to a perplexing question regarding this entire experience. By doing what I did – making it possible for her preference to rehabilitate at home - was I actually depriving her of a personally-needed life experience and/or perspective that a convalescent life-style environment would have provided?

To help gain some insight into the answer to what sounds at first like a contradictory question; I'd like to include some uplifting but still serious subject matter centering on a well-known theory that contributes toward the meaning of life.

To make the difficult and complex as simple as possible I'd like to center on the theory of Karma. Contrary to common belief, the Buddhist term karma; ('cause and effect') is neither good, nor bad, nor ugly – nor is it a 'religious' term. Karma basically has to do with how you handle those issues you bring with you into this life to work out and understand so that you can move forward on your personal spiritual path.

It's common-sense really, no matter what religion you believe in or don't believe in, no matter what your ethnic background or traditions in which you were raised; everyone given the opportunity of life on this plane of existence will experience important personal challenges, decisions and journeys, it's unavoidable. Acknowledgement of this process will allow for the possibility of perfecting ourselves through "thought, word and deed" to further gain awareness and understanding about ourselves and others.

The truth in this is that deep down, most of us strive to be a 'good person'; and the simplest way to achieve that is to treat each person the way you would want to be treated; the old "Golden Rule". With that in mind, we can see how our karma hovers around every move we make and even in the most casual of conversations we speak. We are given choices every day to make easy and hard decisions, if not in action, then in our own minds. Many of the things we say or do are connected to our development as humans toward a spiritual goal whether we are conscious of it or not. Unfortunately these interactions, whether initiated or in a response, tend to originate from our primal human well-spring of the need to be correct, in control, knowledgeable, or in power. Even compliments can sometimes actually be seen as a way of elevating oneself over another. Blatant negativity on the other hand is an obvious act of desperation to belittle anything that does not suit the individual's beliefs and therefore falsely elevates that individual in their mind only. Therein lies the basis for most wars throughout the history on this planet; the belief that there is only 'one way' to perceive things. The fact is; there are as many ways to perceive things that there are people on this planet. The only thing that we all agree on is reality; as reality is based on agreement.

Although there are many, here are two very good examples of "Karma-In-Action" that everyone experiences. One is "Issue Avoidance"; the continual avoidance of important personal issues that keep presenting themselves to you - that's your higher self pointing out your need to address those issues. Granted this process can be difficult, painful, frustrating and annoying but it can also be humbling, joyful, rewarding and spiritually uplifting – it all depends on how honest and how serious you are about dealing with your personal issues. Remember, *that which we resist; persists.*

The other example of "Karma-In-Action" is the theory of the "Absolute Statement". Ever notice how in nearly every movie when the two lovers say to each other, "We have the rest of our lives to be together.", that it's a sure sign in a scene coming up that one of them will die? That's a clear example of what not to say aloud in a universe that challenges your "Absolute Statements". Every time you ignore, avoid or put-off a personal issue or make an absolute statement such as, "I'll never do that!" or any variation thereof, you have just signed-up for it; you just moved that issue to the top of your very own list.

If you're a new soul then you may be too independent in your thinking and laugh all this karma rubbish off - that's fine and as it should be. If you're an old soul then you may have already come to this understanding.

One of my main personal recurring life issues involves "challenging authority" - unjust authority specifically - which I've been doing to varying degrees my entire life. This became such a natural part of me that I never really connected the dots until this 'event'. The reality was that I had experienced numerous and varied incidents that dealt with rebellious personal, as well as altruistic, clashes with 'authority'. And the vast majority of these incidents involved some level of 'legal' involvement.

As an average Baby Boomer I was brought up in a typical "Leave It To Beaver" atmosphere and like Wally and the Beav we did not question authority. Ironically years later "Question Authority" became a classic counter-culture bumper sticker that I've since lived by.

When I was 19 I was in the middle of the sex, drugs and rock and roll youth culture, as nearly most Baby Boomers were to some extent, and I was feeling really good about myself and because of this youthful pride I now realized that I initiated a curse upon myself. One day while at my local beach looking out at the Pacific Ocean, I made an 'Absolute Statement' out loud to the universe that, "I didn't need anyone; no leaders, no god, no institutions, no religions, no one - I could stand alone and take on all comers and prevail." This was more of an outright challenge than a mere absolute statement and only many years later did I realize that I had opened my own Karmic Pandora's Box with that challenge and I have been seriously living and battling the manifested results my entire life! *But then again, apparently that's one of the things that I'm here to learn, understand and resolve; my zealous, overt and rebellious issues regarding unjust authority.*

Therefore it only makes sense that one day I would end up facing the highest court in the land, the Supreme Court, in which to stage a battle for my life. And since I lived my life justly, the situation would require an unjust journey through incredible difficulties toward a confrontation that would force me to develop serious new aspects of understanding and awareness. So ultimately my "Absolute Statement" was not actually a curse, but a blessing, a painful blessing.

What did I learn? Was there a resolution? There are no simple answers. Since this was certainly a culmination of my own life's karmic issues I have to take the obvious and the hidden elements and examine them all carefully; as serious under-standing works on many levels.

Life lessons that are learned too easily are devalued – the more difficult and intense the lesson, the more highly valued. Since my experience certainly qualifies as 'difficult' it is highly valued and I need to gain as much awareness and understanding possible that this situation has created for my benefit.

And even though I went through 'Hell' and am still not out of the fire; I'm personally grateful for this life-lesson opportunity as those of you who have knowledge of prior-life commitments will understand.

One of the most treasured results of these life-lessons is that: *Once your consciousness is raised, it cannot be lowered.*

All of this leads to a classic karmic "what if?" question that a good friend and I have explored over the years, which is; "If you were to see someone about to perform any act of personal, possibly deadly harm and if you were able to prevent it, would you?" The first common-sense reaction and answer would probably be, "Yes." But we realized that by the interaction at an emotional point like that you would now take on some aspect of that person's karma. How is that possible? Well, just normal innocent everyday casual meetings can cause karmic interplay. Any relationship with another living thing creates a meaningful connection whereby our spirits intertwine. To what degree of importance or influence either has on the other depends on the level of "give and take" needed. We wisely concluded that ultimately you should not intercede as we cannot know what they are experiencing or what they *need* to experience. But then again what if that is just what is needed? For you to intercede so you *both* gain the greater shared experience.

So again, what's the answer? The answer is that there are no wrong or bad decisions regarding anything in your life. What may be considered a wrong decision at the time is in fact the catalyst for an opportunity to learn and to achieve a higher level of understanding, experience, awareness and consciousness regarding issues great and small.

Can a 'wrong' decision cause regret? Sure, but regret, as painful as it may be, is just a path not taken. Every minute of every day of your life you have choices of paths to take and decisions to make; whether easy or complicated, safe or dangerous, boring or exciting and everything in-between, in all situations you can only choose one – and then hopefully learn from it.

So other than the possibility of depriving my mother of her own needed karmic experience of life in a convalescent home, were my decisions regarding her healthcare 'wrong'? Well, if based on the preceding concept, definitely not. Instead, quite possibly and more importantly for her it may have been to experience the reality of this *specific 'familial event'* to serve as a last chance opportunity to leave behind those aforementioned petty concerns for deeper awareness, greater understanding and personal growth.

For me, this entire surreal 'event' provided the motivation, and ultimately the opportunity, to write this book with the prime intent to reach as many Boomers as possible who may be facing many of these same senior healthcare issues in order to make the following quote come true; "If this information can prevent even one person from going through what I experienced; then it will have been worth the effort".

THIS IS THE END

My experiences leave me no doubt that our life,
as well as our prior and after life,
is what *we* make it.

Live, Learn and Love to the fullest.

ERW

www.ingramcontent.com/pod-product-compliance
Lightning Source LLC
Chambersburg PA
CBHW072209280526
45788CB00002B/948